Ubaid Amir

Infertility

AF755955

Ubaid Amir

Infertility

LAP LAMBERT Academic Publishing

Imprint

Cover image: www.ingimage.com

Publisher:
LAP LAMBERT Academic Publishing
is a trademark of
Dodo Books Indian Ocean Ltd. and OmniScriptum S.R.L publishing group

120 High Road, East Finchley, London, N2 9ED, United Kingdom
Str. Armeneasca 28/1, office 1, Chisinau MD-2012, Republic of Moldova, Europe
Managing Directors: Ieva Konstantinova, Victoria Ursu
info@omniscriptum.com

Printed at: see last page
ISBN: 978-620-9-05409-9

Acknowledgment

With deep reverence and heartfelt gratitude, I dedicate this acknowledgment to all the teachers who have played an integral role in shaping my journey not just as a student, but as a human being. To express my appreciation in words feels limiting, for the debt I owe to my teachers cannot be measured in language alone. Nonetheless, this space serves as a humble tribute to those noble souls who have illuminated my path with the light of knowledge, encouragement, patience, and values.

From the very beginning of my academic life, I have been blessed to learn under the guidance of extraordinary teachers. At each stage whether in the early classrooms of my childhood, the demanding corridors of high school, or the intellectual halls of higher education—every teacher left a mark on my heart and mind. Each taught me not only facts and theories but also the deeper lessons of life: discipline, integrity, curiosity, empathy, and perseverance.

To my **primary school teachers**, thank you for being the first to ignite my love for learning. You taught me the alphabet, numbers, and the wonders of the world in ways that were fun, gentle, and full of warmth. You were the first to recognize potential in me when I was too young to understand it myself. Your encouragement gave me the confidence to ask questions, to try, and to fail without fear. I still remember the stories you told and the colorful posters you used to make abstract concepts come alive. You created a safe and joyful place for learning, and for that, I will always be grateful.

To my **secondary and high school teachers**, thank you for instilling in me the importance of discipline, responsibility, and critical thinking. These years were some of the most formative in my life. You were the ones who introduced me to the deeper, more complex aspects of the subjects I would come to love. You taught me to organize my thoughts, to analyze problems, and to strive for excellence. But beyond that, you taught me how to cope with failure, how to stand up after setbacks, and how to value hard work over shortcuts. You saw not just a student, but a young person with dreams—and you guided me toward them.

To my **college and university professors**, I owe you a debt I may never fully repay. You challenged me to think beyond the surface, to read deeply, to write critically, and to speak with clarity and conviction. You gave me the tools not only to succeed academically but also to evolve intellectually. Some of you became mentors, shaping not just my understanding of subjects but my entire worldview. In your lectures, I found inspiration; in your office hours, I found guidance; and in your honest feedback, I found growth. You were patient when I faltered, stern when I strayed, and generous with your praise when it was earned. You modeled what it means to pursue knowledge with humility and purpose.

To the **teachers who taught without teaching**, I also extend my heartfelt thanks. Some lessons came not from textbooks but from observing your actions—your patience, your kindness, your dignity in the face of challenges, and your commitment to your work. You showed that teaching is not limited to lectures but can also be expressed through character and conduct. Your actions taught me the values of empathy, respect, and self-discipline. In quiet moments, your example spoke louder than words ever could.

I also wish to acknowledge the **teachers who taught me beyond the walls of classrooms**—those in workshops, seminars, online platforms, and life itself. Many of you never met me personally, yet your words reached me, challenged me, and helped me grow. Your insights, drawn from experience and dedication, contributed immensely to my personal and professional development.

A special acknowledgment must go to the **Unani scholars and mentors** who preserved and passed on a tradition of healing that is both scientific and spiritual. You did more than teach me a medical system; you connected me to centuries of wisdom, compassion, and holistic understanding. Your depth of knowledge, commitment to the roots of Unani medicine, and insistence on integrating theory with practice have inspired me deeply. Under your tutelage, I have come to understand the importance of balance—not only in health but in life. Your mentorship has been a true blessing.

To those teachers who held me accountable when I fell short, thank you. Your firmness helped me realize my potential and reminded me that learning is a responsibility. To those who saw the good in me even when I doubted myself, thank you for believing in me. Your faith has been a source of strength during times of uncertainty. To those who pushed me beyond my comfort zone, thank you for expanding my horizons. You taught me to never settle for mediocrity when excellence is possible.

This acknowledgment would be incomplete without recognizing the **collective spirit of teaching** that transcends individuals. Teaching is more than a profession—it is a calling, a service, and an art. To teach is to give part of oneself so that another may grow, and that is one of the most selfless acts anyone can do. In every corner of the world, teachers continue to shape lives, lift communities, and sow the seeds of future change. I offer this acknowledgment as a tribute to that noble mission.

Lastly, I thank the Divine for blessing me with such extraordinary teachers and for placing me in the care of those who nurtured not only my intellect but my soul.

In closing, to every teacher who ever contributed to my journey, whether through a single word or a lifetime of instruction **thank you**. Your impact is everlasting. Your lessons live on in every word I write, every choice I make, and every step I take.

Ubaid Amir

Index

Dedicated to

Ibrahim

Infertility

1. Introduction

Infertility is a deeply private and ardently challenging medical condition affecting millions of individuals and couples universally. Defined as the incapacity to conceive after 12 months of regular, unprotected sexual contact, infertility is not just a physical issue—it also carries psychological, social, and sometimes cultural consequences. With changing lifestyles, delayed maternity, and increased awareness, infertility has emerged as a significant public health issue.

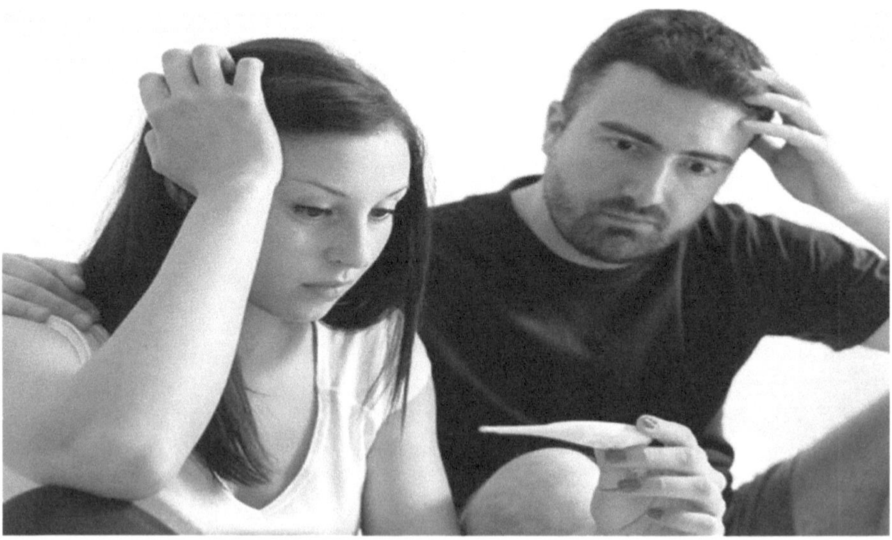

Infertility.

2. Terminology

> ***"If the womb is cold and dry, it will not accept the semen, nor will it nourish it. Likewise, if the semen is weak in heat and spirit, it cannot lead to conception." Ibn Sina.***

"Conception does not occur unless the semen of the man is of proper consistency, warm in temperament, and the uterus of the woman is receptive, warm, and free of obstructions." Galen (Jalinoos).

The amount of both semen and menses are important for fertility potential and whenever either or both are low or minimal, that can cause infertility." Al Razi.

"We should be thinking about it not just as a birth, but a well-being issue." Dr. Giuliano Testa

"I became progressively more interested in infertility ... because ... I became aware of the pain of those who were unable to conceive." Dr. Mike Pawson

"If the temperament of a woman becomes cold, it causes zo'afe jigar"—a liver weakness—leading to impaired reproductive functions and difficulty conceiving."

- Unani medicine—engrained in Greek, Persian, and Arabic traditions—refers to infertility as **'Uqr'**. Classical cradles like *Al-Qānūn fī al-Ṭibb* (Ibn Sīnā) and *Kāmil-us-Ṣanā'* (Majūsi) describe uterine tonics (muqawwi-i-raḥim), aphrodisiacs (muqawwi-i-bah), and ovulation-inducing agents (muwallid-i-manī) for reproductive disorders such as amenorrhea, anovulation, and male weakness.
- These classic texts, compiled by authorities like Hakīm Muḥammad Sharīf Khan and others, offer extensive formulations addressing fertility, including habits, humoral balance (mizāj), and herbal combinations.

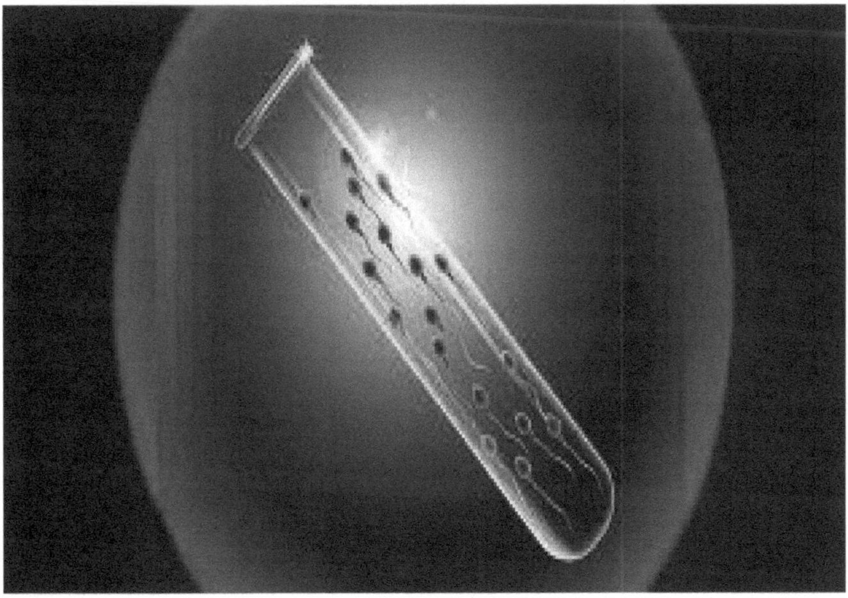

3. Understanding Infertility

Infertility can be categorized into two main types:

- **Primary infertility**: When a person has never conceived despite regular unprotected sex for at least a year.
- **Secondary infertility**: When a person has conceived at least once but is now unable to do so again.

It affects both men and women, and in many cases, it may be due to factors from both partners or remain unexplained despite thorough testing.

According to the World Health Organization (WHO), infertility affects about 15% of reproductive-aged couples globally. This rate varies due to issues like socioeconomic status, access to healthcare, environmental conditions, and cultural beliefs.

4. Unexplained primary infertility

There are so many Unani medicines for treatment of infertility **i.e Safūf Mu‘īn-i-Ḥaml, Ma‘jūn i-Mocharas, Khamīrah Gāozabān Ṣa‘dā, Sharbat Zanjabeel**: administered accordingly. Conception occurred after treatment with some health advise by hakeem. These compounds are said to have uterine tonic and aphrodisiac properties with active constituents like tannins, with anolides, flavonoids and multivitamins.

Unexplained primary infertility (“Uqr nafsī”) in Unani literature is managed using classical formulations grounded in humoral theory and herbal pharmacology. Key formulations include **Safūf Mo‘īn-i-Ḥaml, Ma‘jūn Mocharas**, and powdered herbal blends rich in pharmacologically active constituents

5. Core Herbal Agents & Modes of Action

Across these cases and studies, several key herbs recur:

- **Withania somnifera** (Ashwagandha): supports hormonal balance, antioxidant activity, semen quality.
- **Anogeissus latifolia, Nymphaea alba, Barleria prionitis**: often combined for ovulation induction and uterine tonicity.
- **Mucuna pruriens (Kawach)**: Enhances libido, semen quality, and sperm count.
- **Myristica fragrans (Jaiphal)**: Increases desire and is used in impotence.
- **Zingiber officinale (Zanjabeel)**: Boosts blood flow and strengthens libido.
- **Tribulus terrestris (Gokhru)**: Improves sexual desire and treats male infertility.

•	**Syzygium aromaticum (Laung)**: Enhances sexual stamina and treats premature ejaculation.
•	**Majūn mocharas, Mu'īn-i-Ḥaml, Safūf mocharas, Safūf darchīnī, Majūn Dabidul Ward, Itrifal Shatrta, Majūn Ard Khorma, Majoon Supari Pak**: polyherbal preparations believed to act as uterine tonics (muqawwi-i-raḥim), fertility stimulants, semen enhancers, and libido boosters.

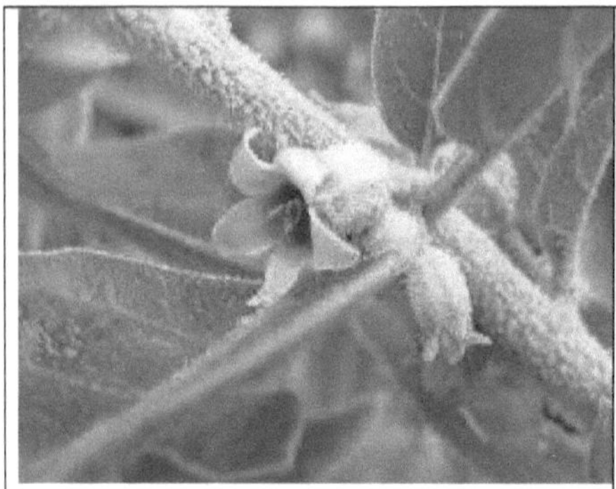

Figure : Withamnia somnifera

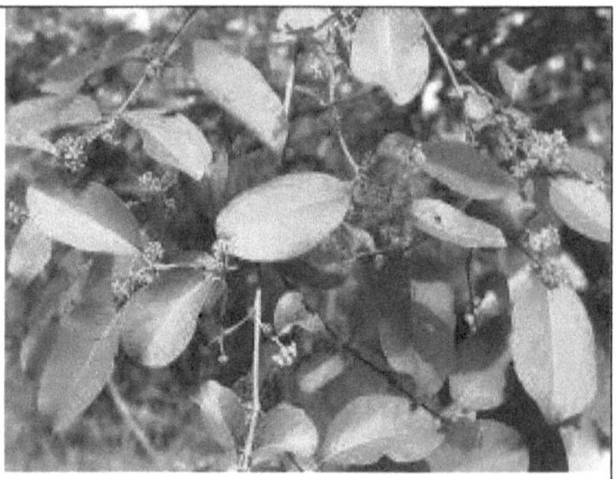

Figure Anogeissus latifolia

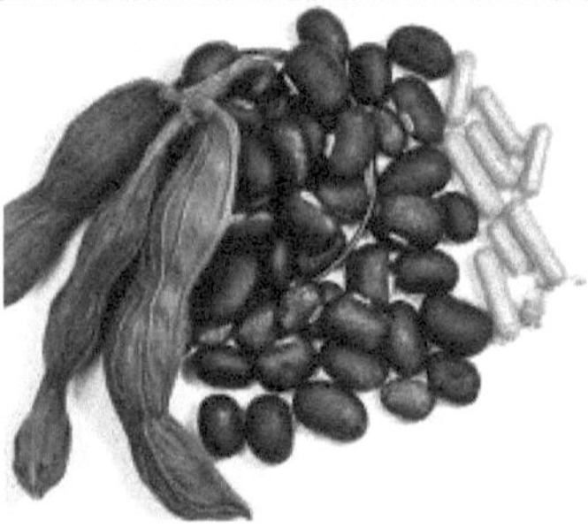

Figure : Mucuna pruriens

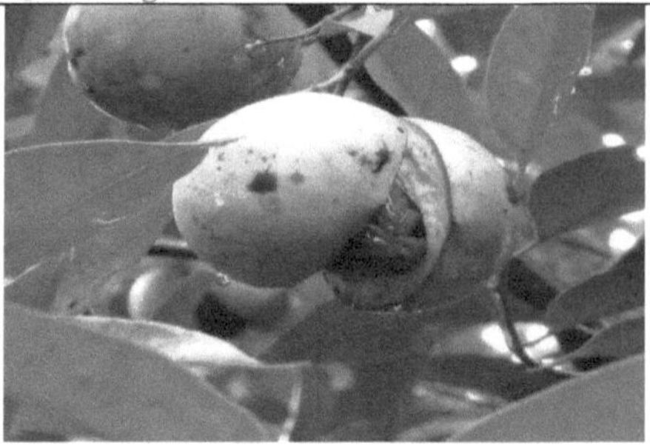

Figure Myristica fragrans

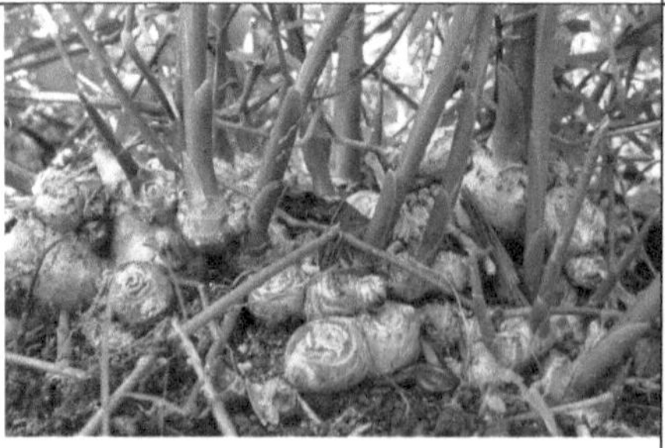

Figure Zingiber officinale

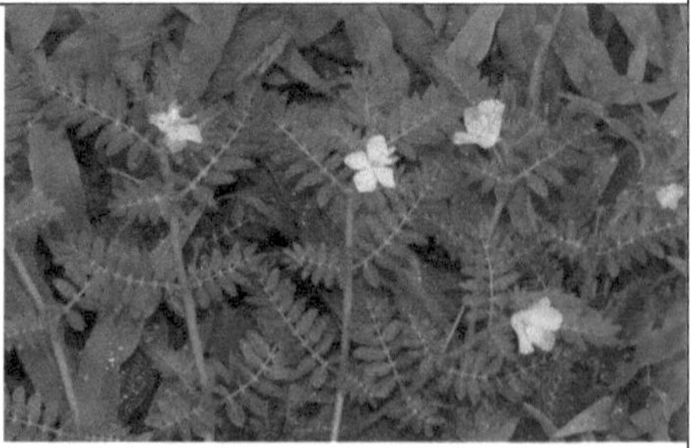

Figure : Tribulus terrestris

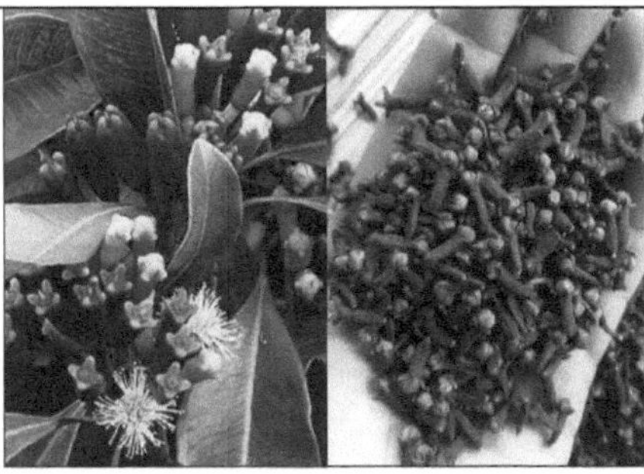

Figure : Syzygium aromaticum

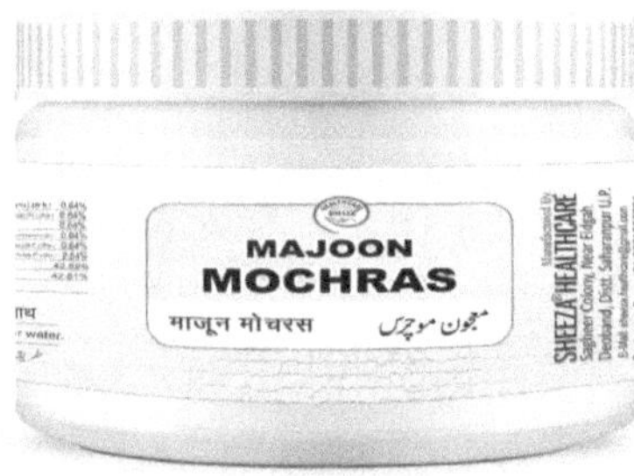

Figure : Majūn mocharas

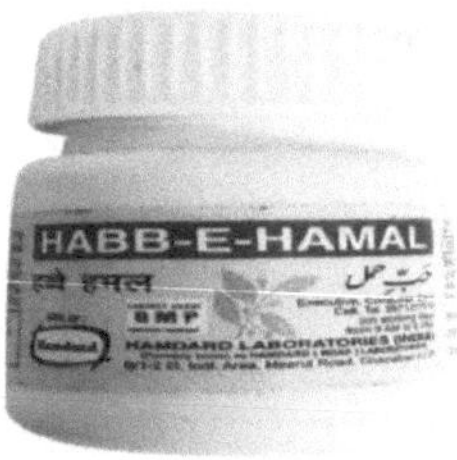

Figure : Habbe Hamal

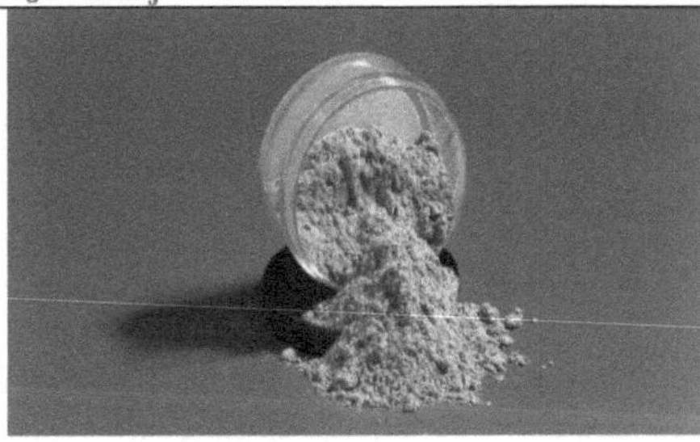

Figure : Safoof Mocharas

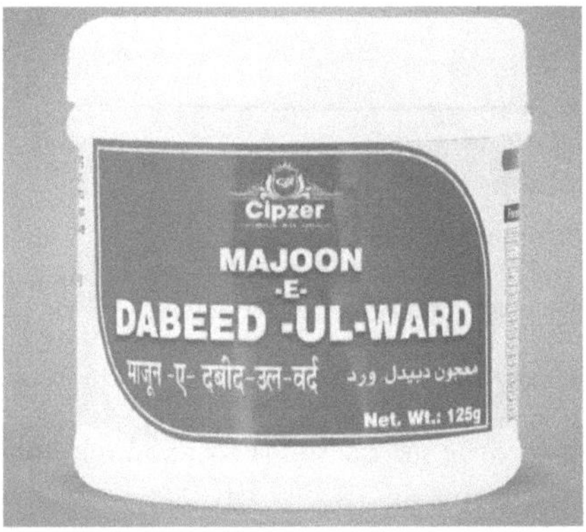

Figure : Majoon Dabidul Ward

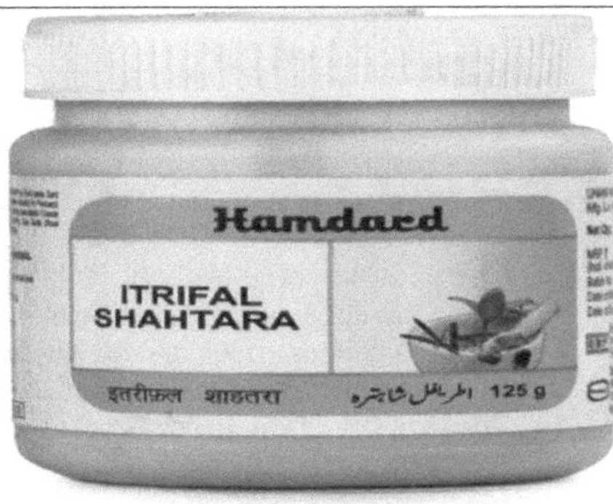

Figure: Itrifal Shatra

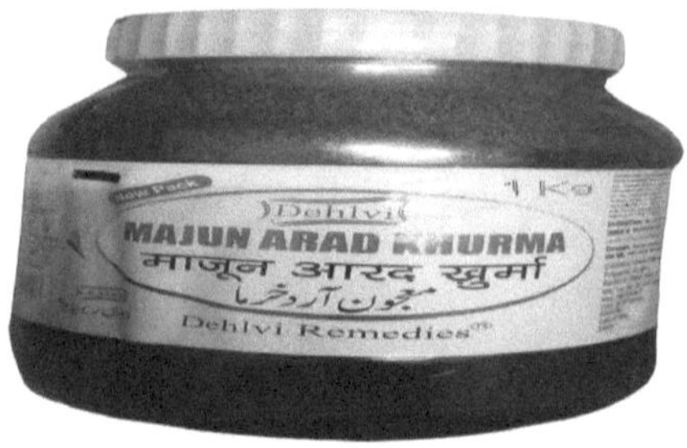

Figure : Majoon Arad Khurma

6. Types of Aphrodisiac Medicines

Unani aphrodisiacs are generally classified into:

1. **Muqawwi-e-Bah**: Enhancers of sexual vigor and libido.
2. **Muwallid-e-Mani**: Agents that help in the formation of semen.
3. **Muqawwi-e-Tanasuliyyah**: Tonics for reproductive organs.
4. **Munzij wa Mukhrij**: Semen-thinning and expelling agents to help in proper ejaculation.

These formulations are thought to contain **steroidal lactones, alkaloids, flavonoids, tannins** and other bioactive constituents thought to enhance folliculogenesis, uterine receptivity, semen quality, or sexual vigor.

7. Causes of Infertility

Female Factors

1. **Ovulation Disorders**
    - These account for approximately 25% of female infertility cases.
    - Conditions include polycystic ovary syndrome (PCOS), hypothalamic dysfunction, premature ovarian insufficiency, and hyperprolactinemia.
2. **Fallopian Tube Damage or Blockage**
    - Often caused by pelvic inflammatory disease, endometriosis, or previous surgeries.
    - Tubal issues prevent the sperm from reaching the egg or the fertilized egg from reaching the uterus.
3. **Endometriosis**
    - This occurs when uterine tissue grows outside the uterus, causing inflammation and scarring, which may block fallopian tubes or affect ovarian function.

4. **Uterine or Cervical Abnormalities**
    - Congenital anomalies, fibroids, or cervical stenosis can interfere with implantation or sperm transport.
5. **Age-Related Factors**
    - Female fertility significantly declines after age 35 due to a reduction in the quantity and quality of eggs.

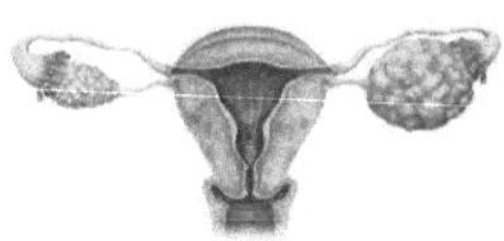

Figure : PCOD

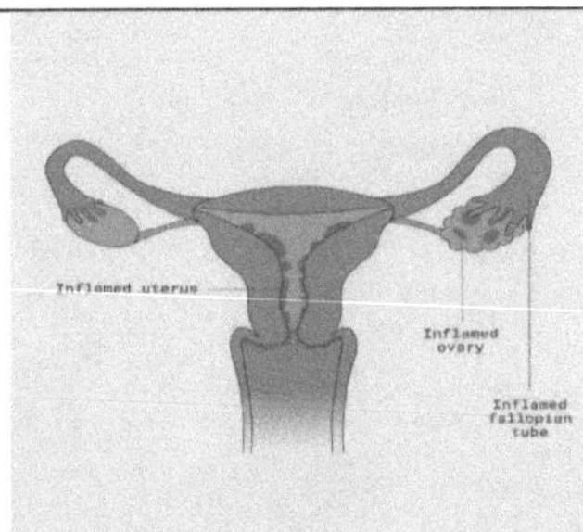

Figure : PID

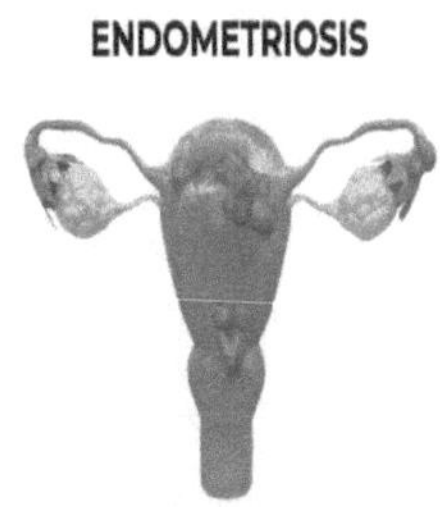

Figure : Endometriosis

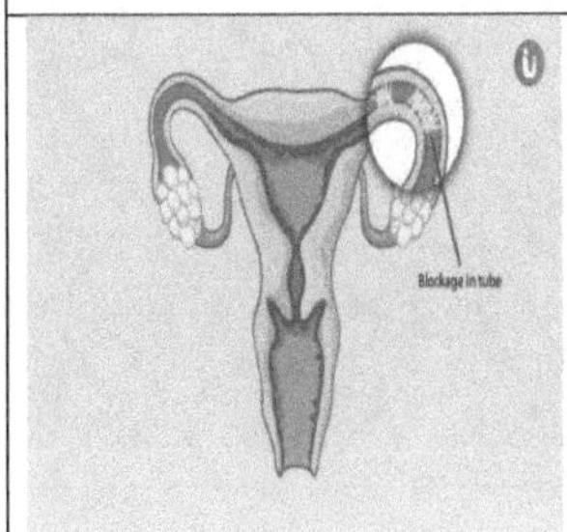

Figure : Tubal Blockage

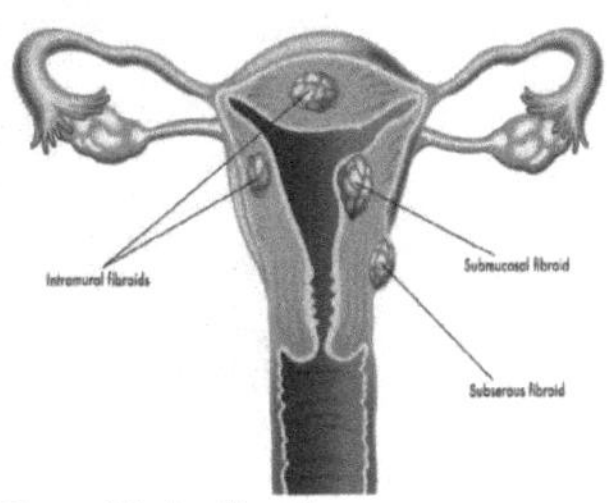

Figure: Uterine fibroid

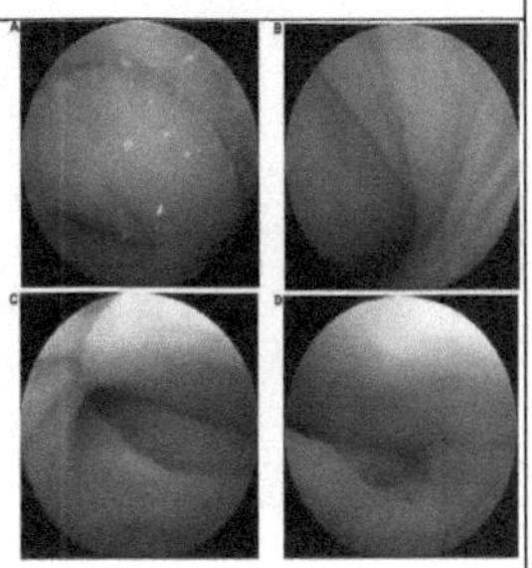

cervial stensois

Male Factors

1. **Sperm Production Disorders**
   - Low sperm count, poor motility, or abnormal morphology can significantly impair fertility.
   - Causes include genetic factors, infections (e.g., mumps orchitis), varicocele, or hormonal imbalances.
2. **Obstruction of Sperm Transport**
   - Vas deferens blockage or absence, due to infections or congenital conditions like cystic fibrosis, can prevent sperm from being ejaculated.
3. **Ejaculation Disorders**
   - Retrograde ejaculation or premature ejaculation can hinder fertilization.
4. **Lifestyle and Environmental Factors**
   - Excessive alcohol consumption, smoking, exposure to toxins, obesity, and certain medications may impair sperm function.

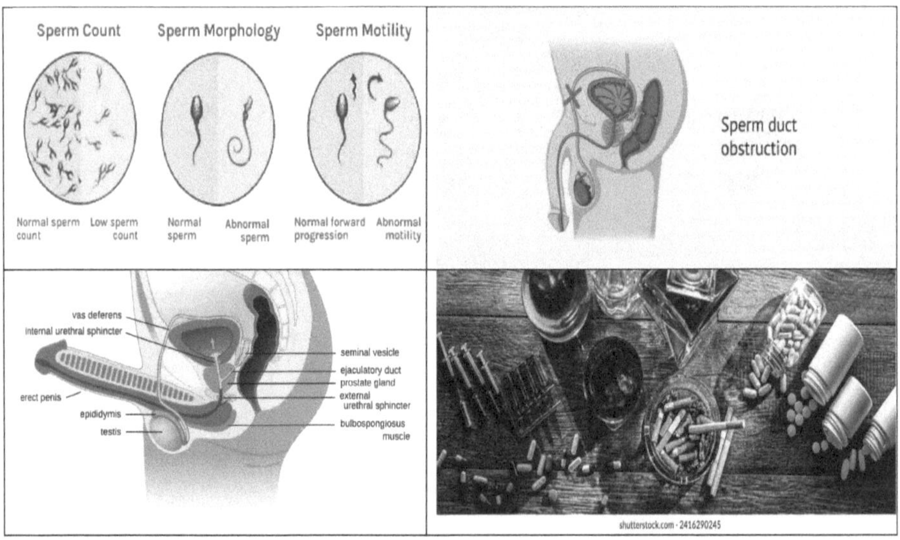

Combined and Unexplained Factors

In approximately 20% of couples, both partners have fertility issues. In 10–15% of cases, no clear cause is identified, known as unexplained infertility. These cases can be particularly frustrating and emotionally taxing for couples.

8. Causes of Infertility in Unani Literature (Asbāb-e-'Uqr)

In Unani medicine, infertility is known as **'Uqr** and is understood as the inability to conceive due to **imbalance in temperament (Mizāj)**, **humoral disturbances**, and **structural or functional ailments** of the reproductive organs in men or women. The Unani concept of infertility is holistic, participating physical, emotional, and ecological factors.

General Causes (Asbāb-e-'Āmmah)

These are systemic or general causes affecting fertility in both sexes:

1. **Imbalance of Mizāj (Temperament)**
   - According to Unani system of medicine each organ has a natural temperament. A deviation (either excessive hot, cold, oist, or dry) can damage reproductive function.
   - **Cold and dry Mizāj** of the uterus or semen leads to reduced fertility.
2. **Disturbed Akhlāṭ (Humors)**
   - Unani identifies four humors: **Dam (blood)**, **Balgham (phlegm)**, **Safrā' (yellow bile)**, and **Sawdā' (black bile)**.
   - **Dominance of Balgham (cold and moist)** or **Sawdā' (cold and dry)** can spoil ovulation or sperm production.
3. **Weakness of Tabi'at (Vital force)**
   - If the body's normal self-healing power is deteriorated, it cannot support reproductive functions properly.
4. **Inadequate Ghidhā' (Nutrition)**
   - Poor diet indicate to **insufficient production of healthy blood**, which is required for forming semen or maturing eggs.

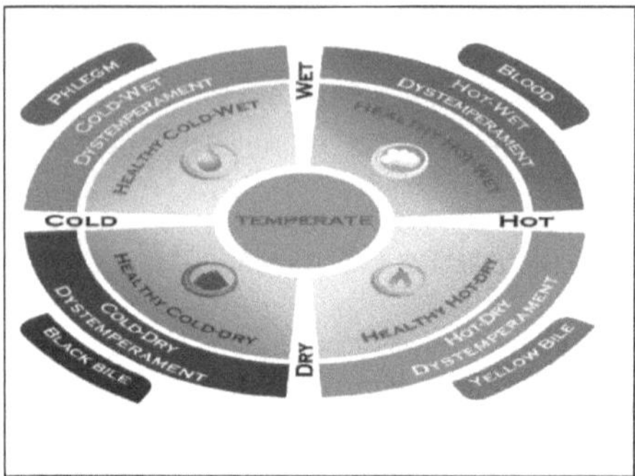
PHLEGM
COLD-WET
DYSTEMPERAMENT
HEALTHY COLD-WET
WET
HOT-WET
DYSTEMPERAMENT
BLOOD
HEALTHY HOT-WET
COLD
TEMPERATE
HOT
HEALTHY COLD-DRY
COLD-DRY
DYSTEMPERAMENT
BLACK BILE
DRY
HEALTHY HOT-DRY
HOT-DRY
DYSTEMPERAMENT
YELLOW BILE

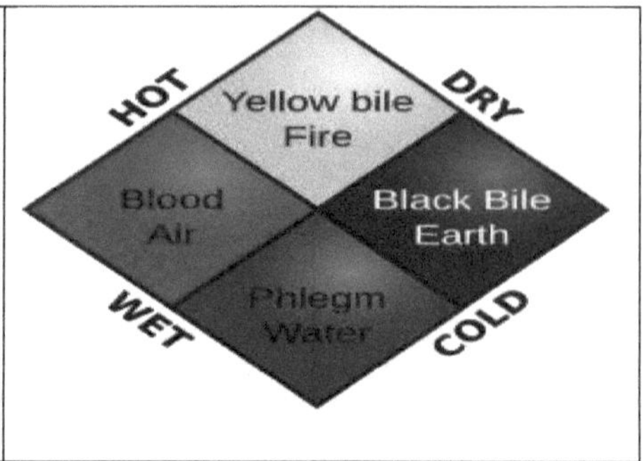
HOT
DRY
Yellow bile
Fire
Blood
Air
Black Bile
Earth
Phlegm
Water
WET
COLD

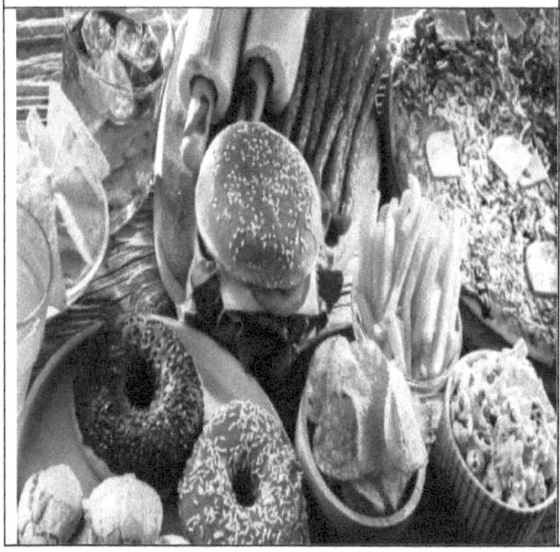

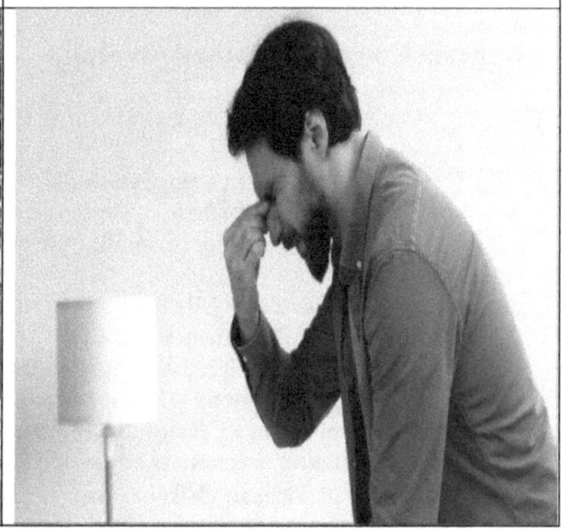

Causes in Females (Asbāb-e-'Uqr fī Nisā')

Unani scholars recognize the following major causes of infertility in women:

1. **Zo'f-e-Raḥim (Uterine Weakness)**
    - A uterus with weak musculature or improper temperament cannot support conception.
2. **Sūdād-e-Raḥim (Uterine Obstruction)**
    - Accumulation of abnormal phlegmatic or melancholic humors in the uterus can block sperm passage or implantation. That can leads to develop sexual problems.
3. **Shiddat-e-Harārat (Excessive Heat)**
    - Causes dryness of the uterus, hampering egg fertilization or implantation.
4. **Buroodat wa Yubūsat (Coldness and Dryness)**
    - A uterus with cold and dry temperament cannot support conception.
5. **Qillat-e-Manī al-Mar'a (Low Female Semen)**
    - In Unani, both men and women are believed to contribute semen; inadequate or poor-quality female semen prevents fertilization.
6. **Ikhtilāl-e-'Ādat al-Tamth (Menstrual Irregularities)**
    - Scanty, irregular, or absent periods (I'tidāl-e-Tamth) prevent the proper maturation of reproductive matter.
7. **Amrāz-e-Raḥim (Diseases of the Uterus)**
    - Includes inflammation, ulcers, tumors, or displacement of the uterus.

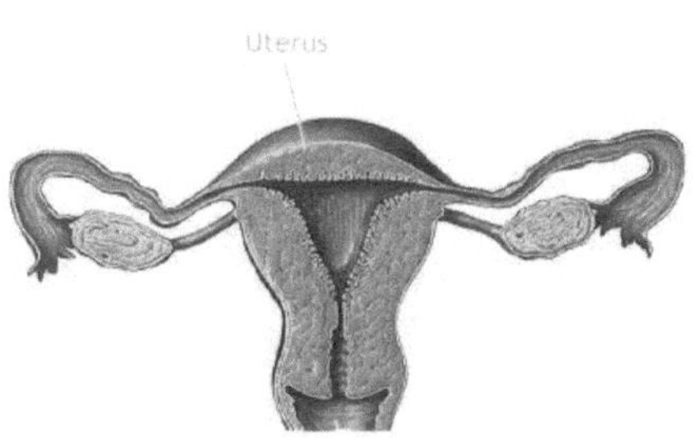

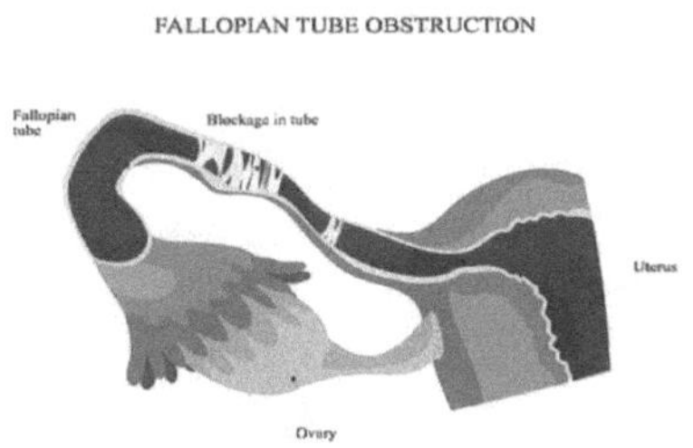

Causes in Males (Asbāb-e-'Uqr fī Rijāl);

1. **Zo'f-e-Bah (Sexual Debility)**
    - Weak sexual power due to general debility, stress, or overindulgence in sexual activity.
2. **Qillat-e-Manī (Low Semen Volume)**
    - Deficiency in semen quantity or quality; sometimes due to humoral imbalances.
3. **Sūdād-e-Mawād (Obstruction in Reproductive Channels)**
    - Obstruction of seminal passages due to phlegm, thick humors, or infections.
4. **Ghair Mutashakkil Manī (Non-Formed Semen)**
    - Semen without proper consistency or form, lacking ability to fertilize.
5. **Imtila' (Fullness of Humors)**
    - Excess of blood or phlegm leading to sluggishness or blockage of reproductive function.
6. **Harārat-e-Kazība (False Heat)**
    - Heat caused by inflammation, not vitality—may lead to ejaculation without fertility.
7. **I'lāl al-A'ḍā' al-Tanasuliyya (Diseases of Sexual Organs)**
    - Includes infections, trauma, varicocele, or malformations of the penis/testes.

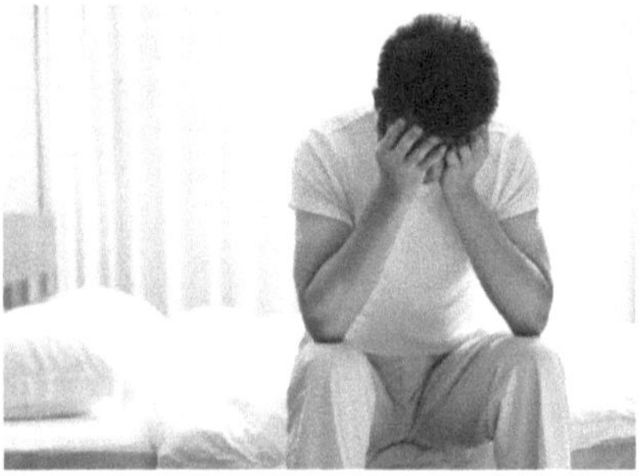

Figure Sexual Debility

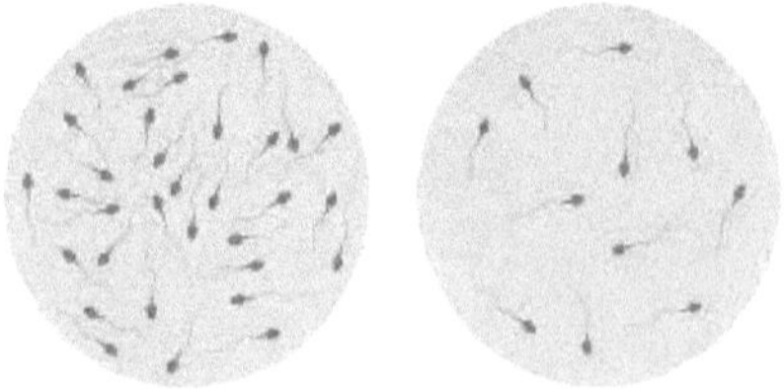

Figure low sperm count

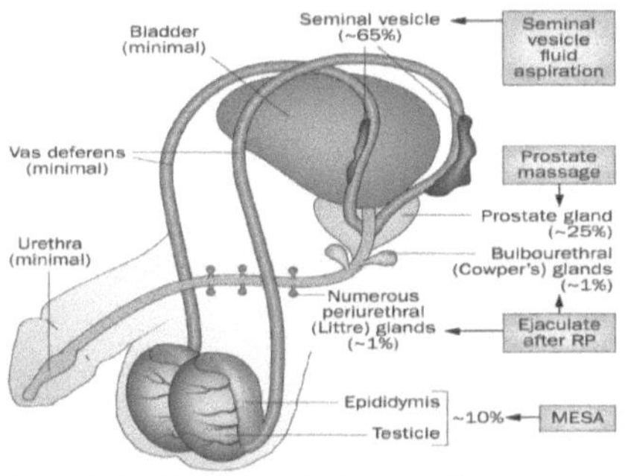

Figure: Obstruction of reproductive channel.

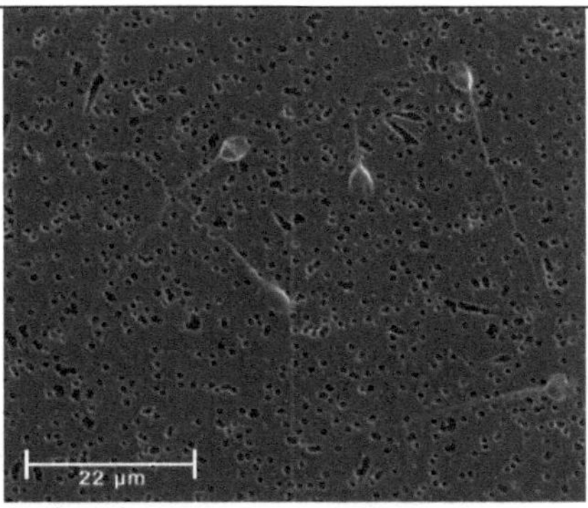

Non formed sperm

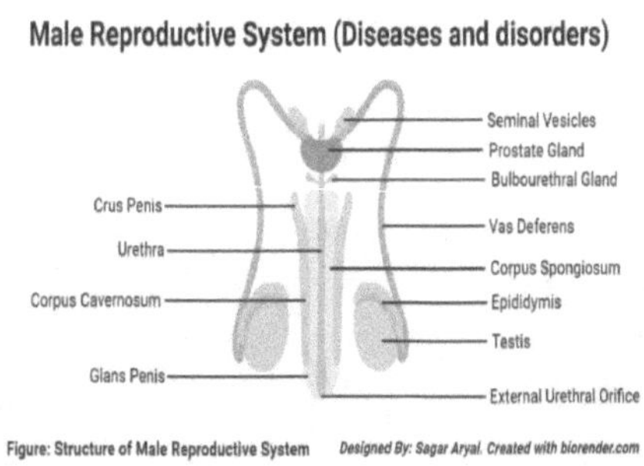

Figure : Diseases of male reproductive system

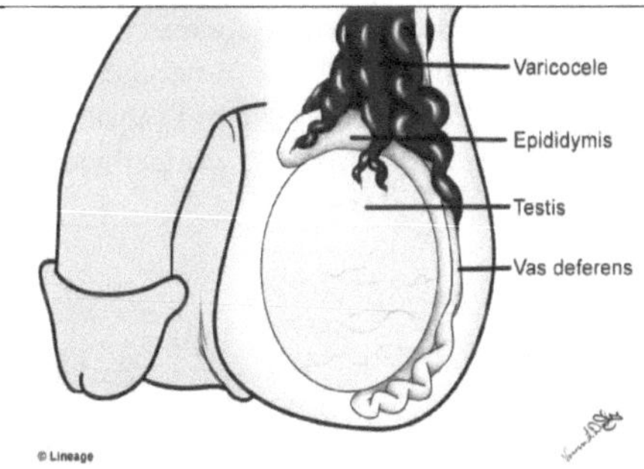

Psychological and Lifestyle Factors

Unani physicians like Ibn Sina accredited mental and emotional health in reproductive well-being.

- **Khauf (Fear), Gham (Depression), Hamm (Anxiety)** – can weaken Tabi'at and reduce sexual desire and fertility.
- **Overeating, lack of exercise, excessive coitus** – considered causes of Zo'f-e-Bah.

9. Diagnosis of Infertility

Diagnosing infertility typically involves both partners and includes the following:

For Women:

- **Ovulation testing**: Hormonal blood tests and tracking menstrual cycles.
- **Imaging tests**: Pelvic ultrasounds, hysterosalpingography (HSG), and laparoscopy.
- **Ovarian reserve testing**: Evaluates the quantity and quality of eggs.
- **Thyroid function and prolactin levels**: To rule out hormonal imbalances.

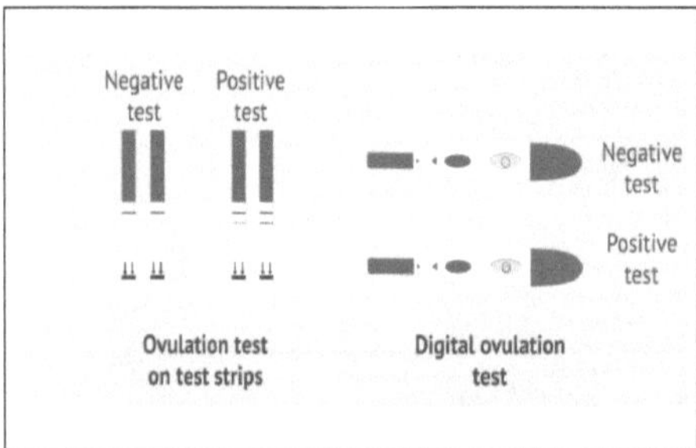

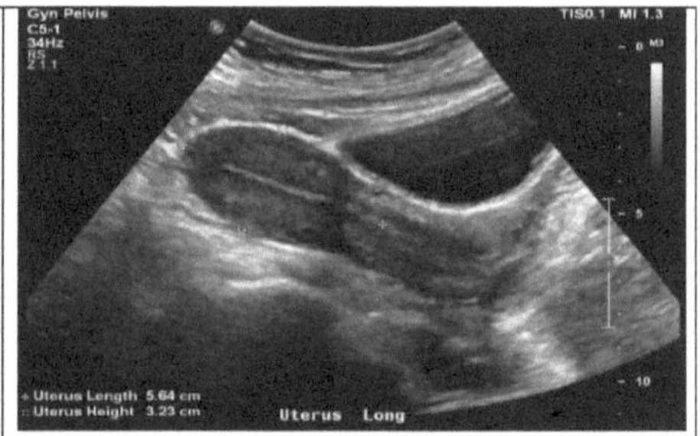

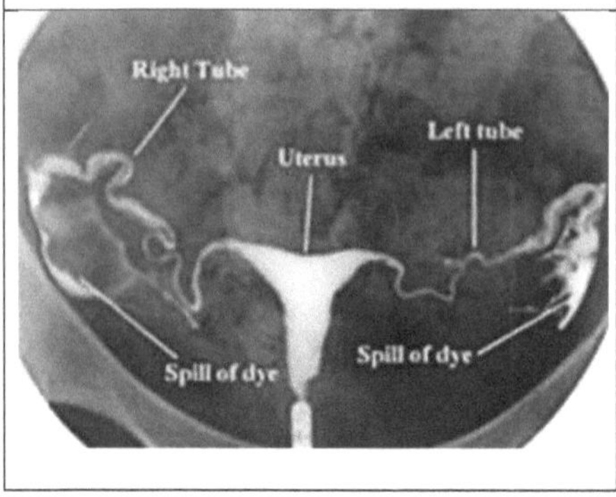

Biochemical test	Normal reference range	Group I (mean ± SD)	Group II (mean ± SD)
T3 (ng/mL)	0.9-1.95	0.98 ± 0.18	1.81 ± 0.22
T4 (ng/dL)	4.4-12.5	9.12 ± 0.96	5.16 ± 0.71
TSH (µIU/L)	0.40-4.5	7.11 ± 1.91	3.28 ± 2.11
Prolactin (ng/mL)	<25	41.62 ± 20.2	22.36 ± 15.6

For Men:

- **Semen analysis**: Assesses sperm count, motility, and shape.
- **Hormonal testing**: Testosterone and other hormone levels.
- **Scrotal ultrasound**: Detects varicocele or other abnormalities.
- **Genetic testing**: If there's no sperm in the semen (azoospermia), genetic issues might be suspected.

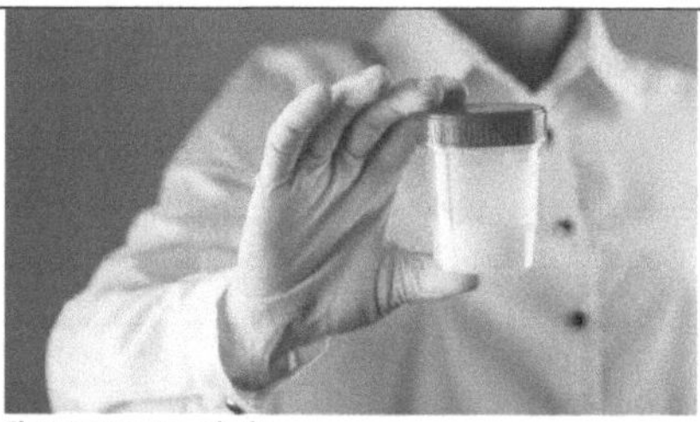

Figure semen analysis

Typical total testosterone levels in adults	
(20-24 years old)	409-558 ng/dL
(25-29 years old)	413-575 ng/dL
(30-34 years old)	359-498 ng/dL
(35-39 years old)	352-478 ng/dL
(40-44 years old)	350-473 ng/dL

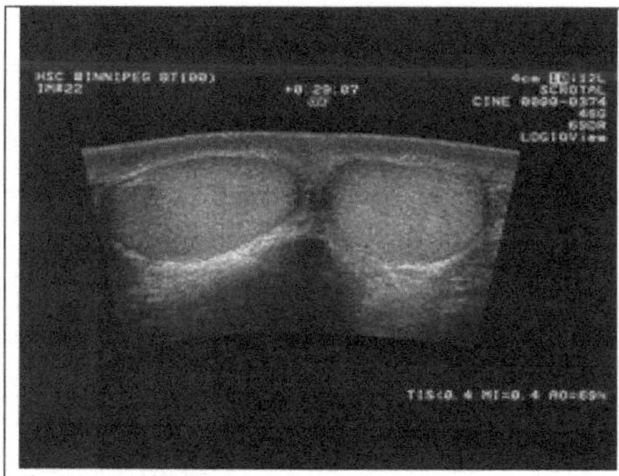

Figure: scrotal USG

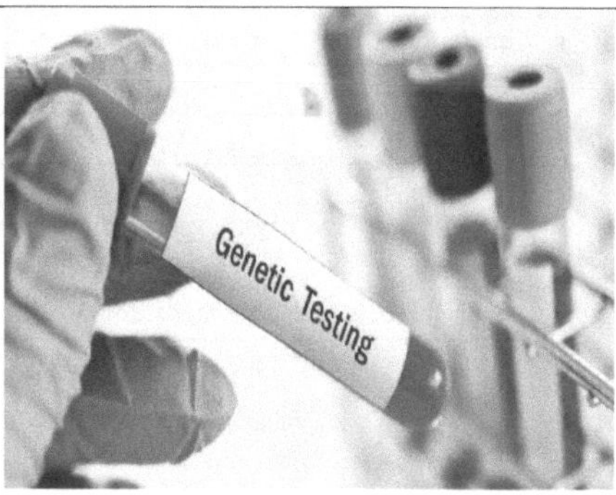

Figure: genetic testing

10. Diagnosis of Infertility in Unani.

In **Unani medicine**, infertility is diagnosed based on traditional concepts entrenched in **humoral theory**, **temperament (Mizaj)**, and the functional integrity of organs responsible for reproduction. Unlike modern medicine, Unani diagnosis includes physical, psychological, dietary, and environmental factors also.

1. History Taking (Riwayat-e-Marid)

• Duration and type of infertility (primary or secondary)
• Menstrual history in females
• Sexual performance and history in males
• Lifestyle, diet, emotional state, stress
• Previous illnesses or infections
• Habits such as smoking, alcohol

2. Temperament Assessment (Tashkhis-e-Mizaj)

• Each person has a **mizaj** (temperament): hot, cold, moist, or dry.
• Reproductive health depends on a **balanced mizaj**.
• For example:

Cold and dry temperament → weak semen or poor ovulation.
Hot and dry temperament → inflammation or uterine dryness.

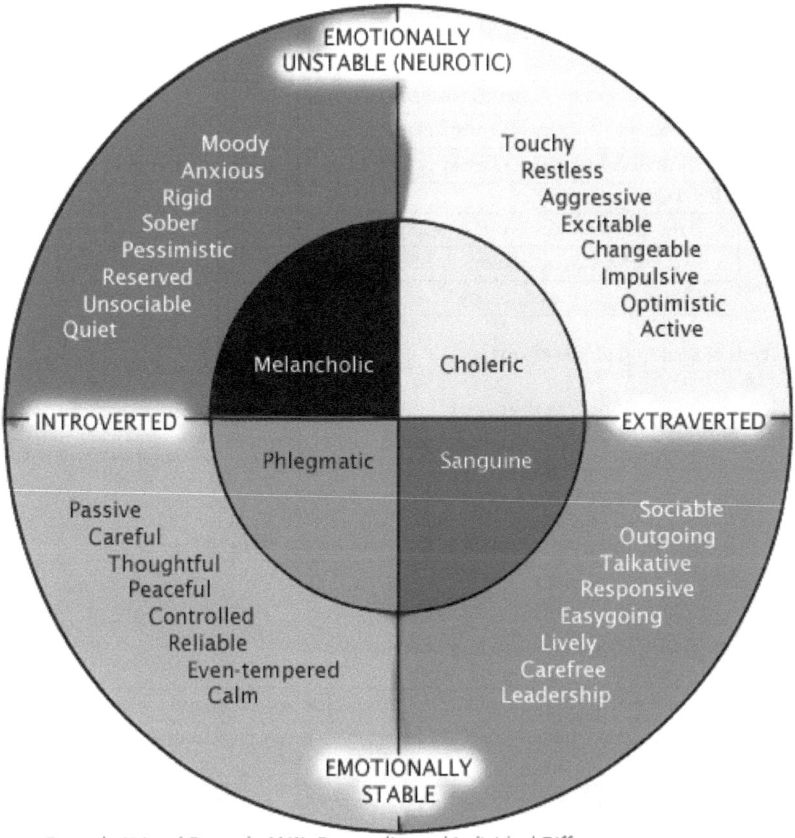

Eysenck, H.J and Eysenck, M.W. *Personality and Individual Differences.* Plenum Publishing, 1958.

3. Examination of Reproductive Organs

- **For males:**

○ Quality, quantity, and consistency of semen.
○ Presence of varicocele, testicular atrophy
○ Sexual desire and performance (linked to Hararat-e-Ghariziyah or innate heat)

- **For females:**

○ Uterine condition (womb warmth, structure).
○ Vaginal discharge (color, smell, consistency).
○ Menstrual cycle regularity.

4. Analysis of Semen (Fahm-e-Mani)

- Evaluated based on four characteristics:

▪ **Rang (Color)**: white or off-white is normal
▪ **Raiha (Smell)**: semen should have a specific musky smell
▪ **Lazajat (Viscosity)**: moderate stickiness
▪ **Miqdar (Quantity)**: sufficient for fertilization

5. Evaluation of Uterus and Menses (Rahim & Haiz)

• Warmth and moisture are essential for the uterus to accept sperm.
• Menstrual disorders (amenorrhea, dysmenorrhea, excessive bleeding) are common causes.
• Cold or dry uterus common cause of infertility.

6. Pulse Diagnosis (Nabz Shanasi)

• Pulse characteristics indicate imbalance in temperament
• Helps determine general and reproductive health.

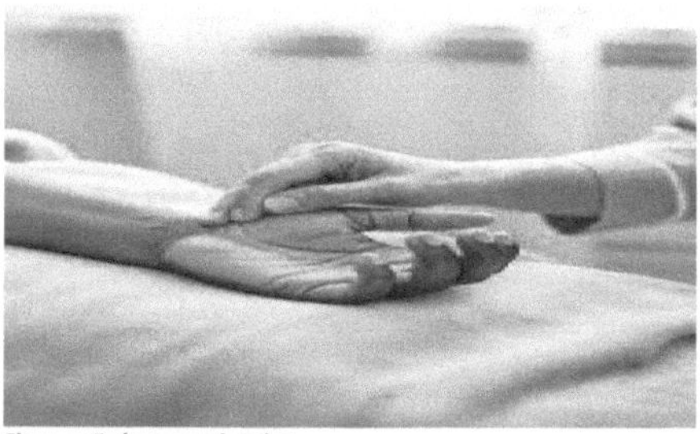

Figure : Pulse examination

7. Urine Examination (Baul Shanasi)

- Color, consistency, and sediments of urine give insights into organ health and systemic imbalances.

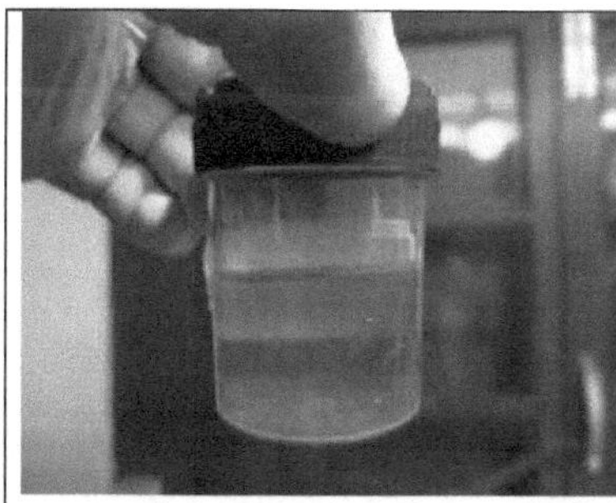

Figure: Urine Examination

Common Causes of Infertility in Unani.

Male Causes	Female Causes
Su-e-Mizaj (imbalanced temperament)	Cold & dry uterus (Baroodat wa Yubusat)
Weakness of seminal fluid	Obstruction in fallopian tubes

Male Causes	Female Causes
Varicocele	Irregular or absent menstruation
Excessive coitus or masturbation	Excess uterine discharge
Malnutrition	General body weakness (I'ya)

Tools and Techniques Used.

• Mizaj assessment (questionnaires, physical signs)
• Semen testing (traditional methods)
• Pulse and urine examination
• Manual pelvic exam
• Inquiry into psychological and dietary factor

11. Treatment of Infertility

Infertility treatment depends on the underlying cause, duration of infertility, age of the partners, and personal preferences. Options include medical, surgical, and assisted reproductive techniques.

Medical Treatments

• **Fertility Drugs**: Medications like clomiphene citrate, letrozole, or gonadotropins stimulate ovulation in women.
• **Hormonal Therapies**: For men and women with hormonal imbalances.
• **Treatment of Underlying Conditions**: Managing PCOS, thyroid disorders, or infections.

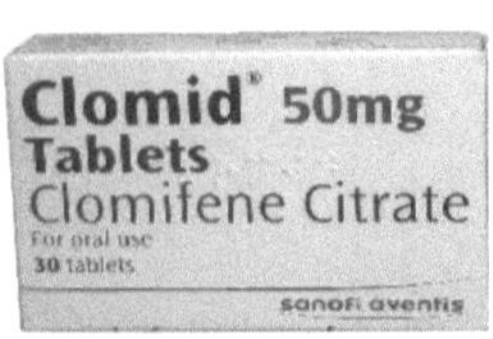

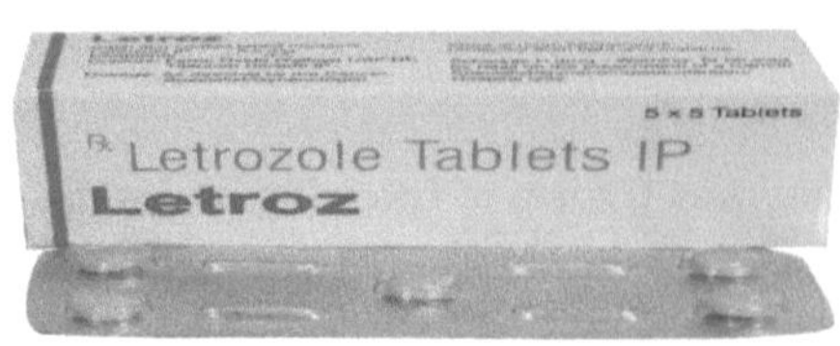

Surgical Treatments

- **Laparoscopy or Hysteroscopy**: To remove endometrial tissue, fibroids, or polyps.
- **Tubal Surgery**: To unblock or repair damaged fallopian tubes.
- **Varicocele Repair**: In men, to improve sperm production.

Assisted Reproductive Technologies (ART)

1. **Intrauterine Insemination (IUI)**: Sperm is directly placed into the uterus around the time of ovulation.

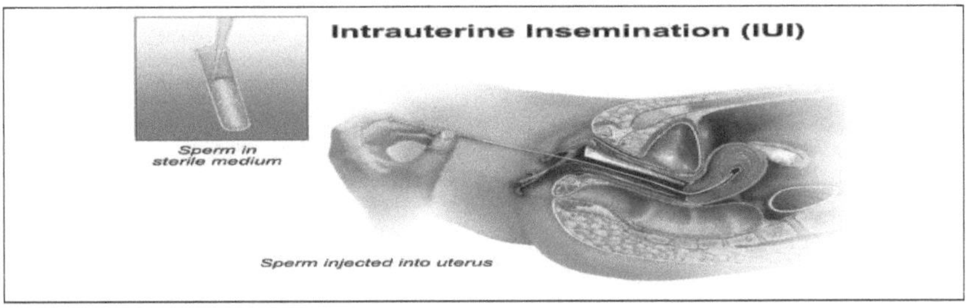

2. **In Vitro Fertilization (IVF)**:
   - Eggs are retrieved and fertilized with sperm in a lab.
   - The resulting embryo is implanted into the uterus.
   - IVF has become a widely used and effective method, although success rates vary based on age and clinic.

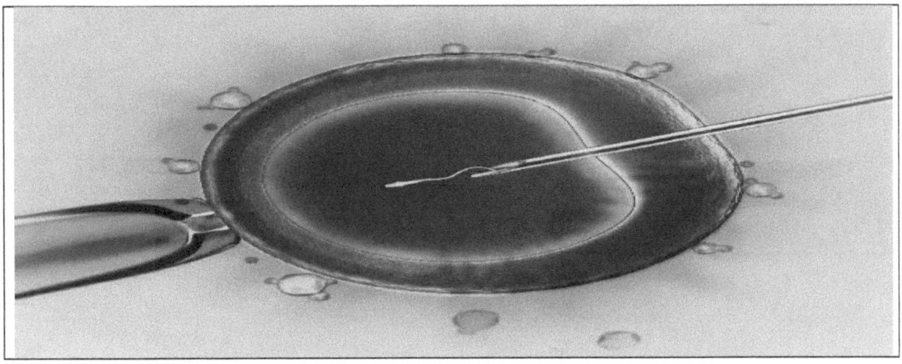

3. **Intra-cytoplasmic Sperm Injection (ICSI)**:
   - A single sperm is injected directly into the egg.
   - Commonly used when male infertility is the primary issue.

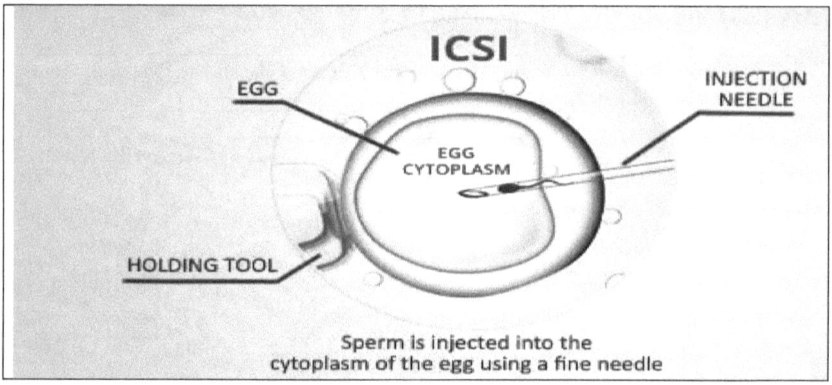

4. **Donor Eggs or Sperm**:
   - Used when one partner is unable to produce viable gametes.

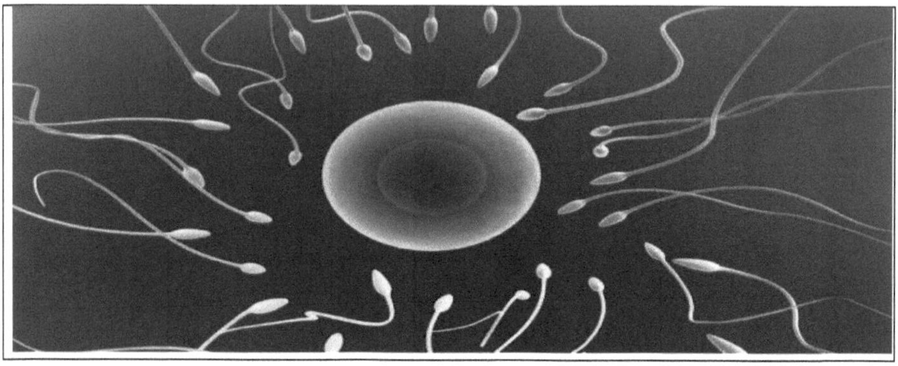

5. **Surrogacy and Gestational Carriers**:
   - Options for women who cannot carry a pregnancy due to uterine issues or health conditions.

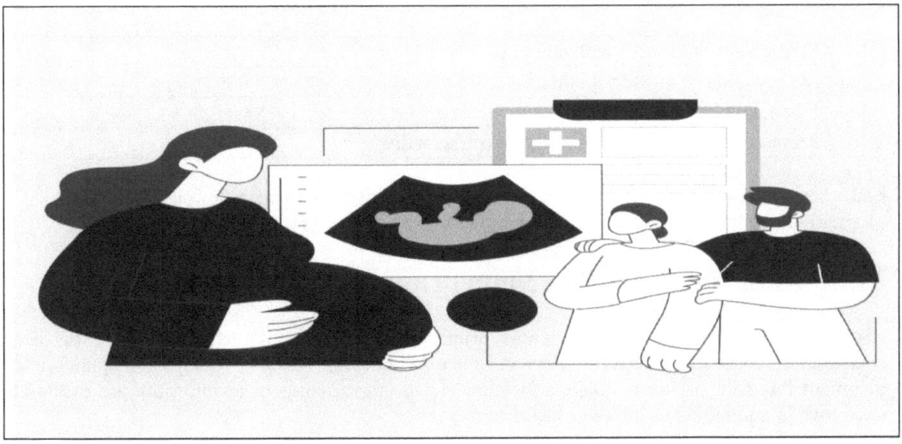

6. **Fertility Preservation**:
   - Egg, sperm, or embryo freezing is increasingly used for individuals undergoing cancer treatment or delaying parenthood.

Psychological and Emotional Impacts

Infertility often triggers a range of emotional responses such as guilt, anger, sadness, and anxiety. Couples may experience relationship strain, sexual dysfunction, and social isolation. Women, in particular, may feel societal pressure and stigma in certain cultures where motherhood is deeply tied to identity.

Support from counseling, support groups, and open communication can play a critical role in managing these emotional challenges. Mental health support should be an integral part of fertility treatment plans.

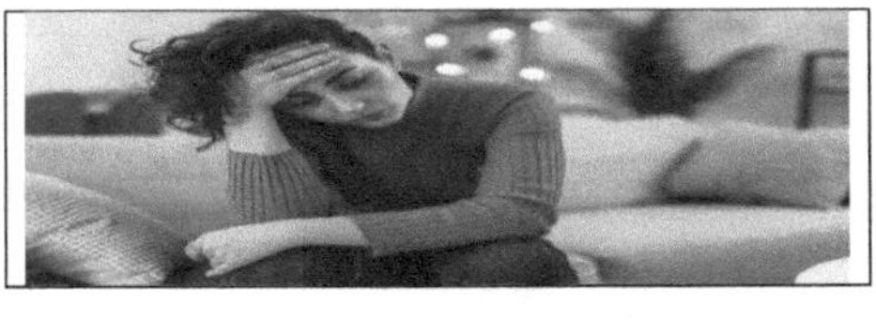

Social and Cultural Implications

In many cultures, especially in developing regions, infertility can lead to profound social consequences, including:

• Stigmatization or marginalization, particularly of women.
• Marital discord or even divorce.
• Financial strain from costly treatments.
• Pressure to seek traditional or unproven remedies.

Educating societies about infertility as a medical issue rather than a moral or personal failing is essential to combat stigma and improve access to care.

Male Infertility and Misconceptions

Historically, infertility has been viewed primarily as a "woman's issue," even with men contributing to 40–50% of infertility cases. This misconception results in delays in diagnosis and treatment for male partners. Public education and destigmatizing male infertility are essential steps toward equitable reproductive healthcare.

Advancements and Ethical Considerations

Modern science has greatly advanced the diagnosis and treatment of infertility, but these developments also raise ethical, legal, and societal questions:

• Who has access to fertility treatment?
• Should there be age or financial limits?
• What are the implications of selecting embryos based on genetic traits?
• How should unused embryos be managed?

These concerns highlight the importance of ethical guidelines and regulatory frameworks in reproductive medicine.

Prevention and Lifestyle Considerations

While not all causes of infertility are preventable, certain lifestyle changes can reduce risk:

• Avoiding smoking, excessive alcohol, and illicit drug use.
• Maintaining a healthy weight.
• Managing stress.
• Avoiding exposure to environmental toxins.
• Timely screening and treatment of sexually transmitted infections.

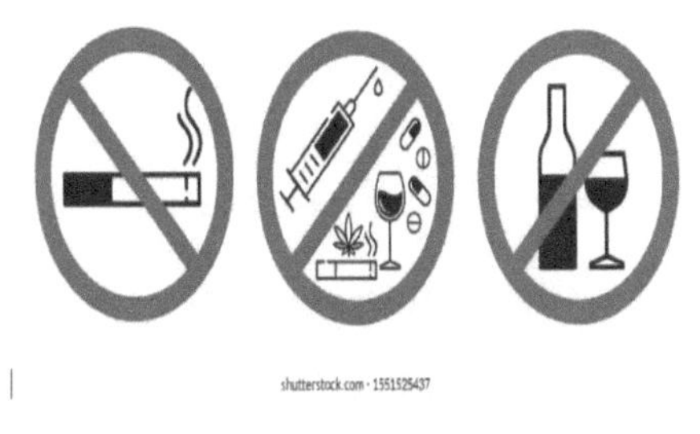

shutterstock.com · 1551525437

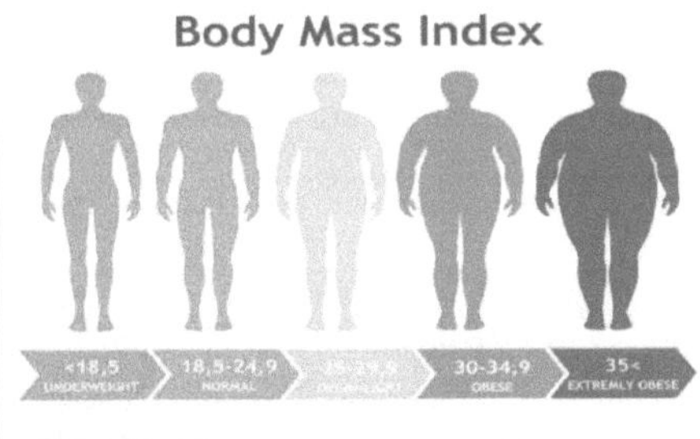

Body Mass Index
<18,5
UNDERWEIGHT
18,5-24,9
NORMAL
30-34,9
OBESE
35<
EXTREMLY OBESE

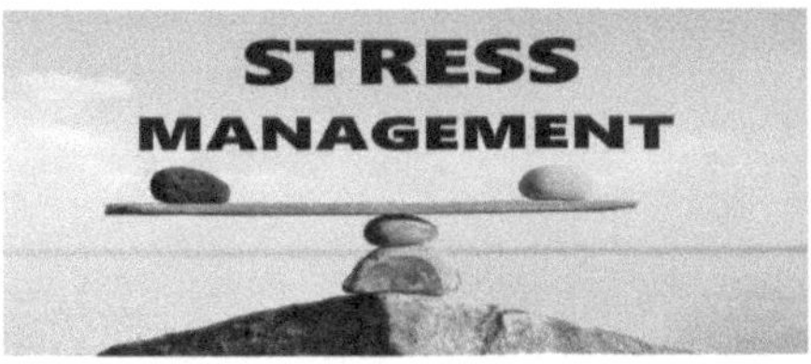

STRESS
MANAGEMENT

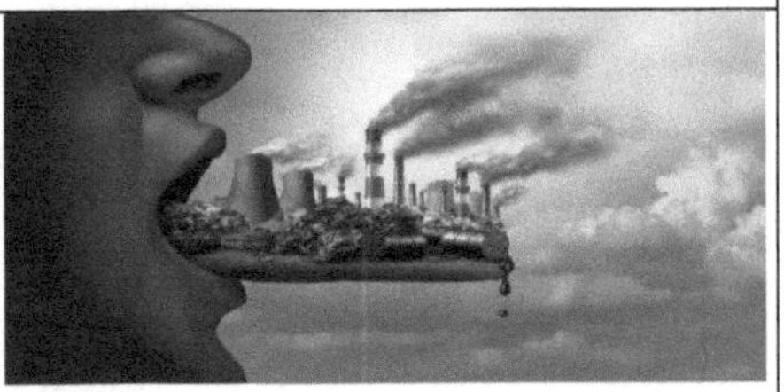

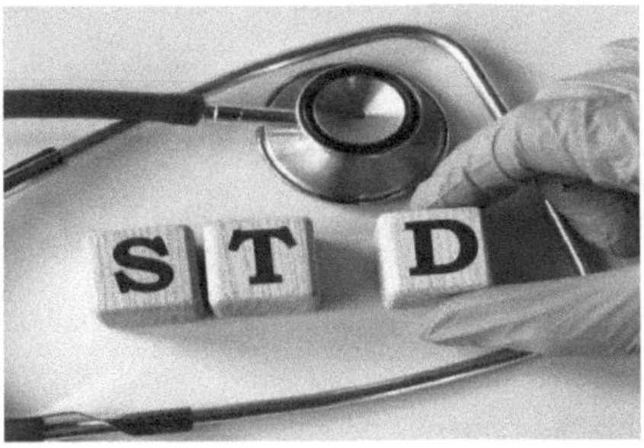

S T D

Unani Principles (Usool) in Treating 'Uqr'

1. Tazkiyah and Imala: (Detoxification and Cleansing)

- **Fasd** (venesection) and **Irsaal-e-Alaq** (leech therapy) are used to purge excess or morbid humors that may impair fertility.
- **Steam baths (Hammam)** aid in toxin elimination through perspiration and enhance circulation.

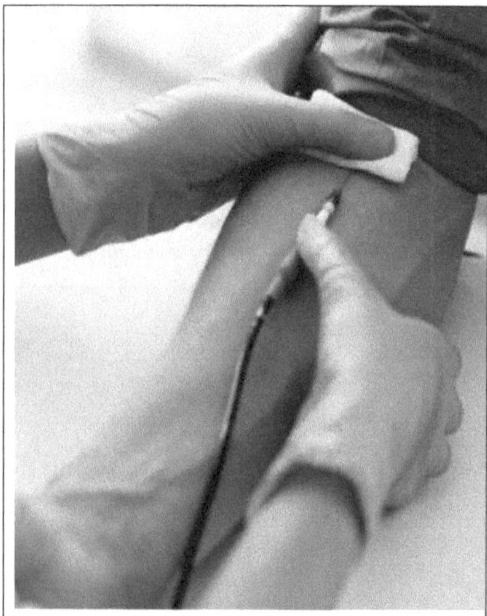

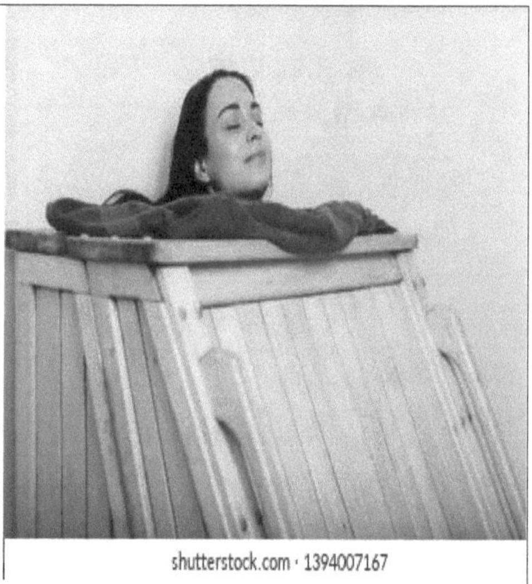

2. Ilaj-bil-Tadbir: Regimens for Health Balance

• Personalized **diet therapy**
• moderate **exercise**
• Stress reduction
• **Massage therapies** such as **Marma** are prescribed to harmonize bodily systems and enhance reproductive readiness.

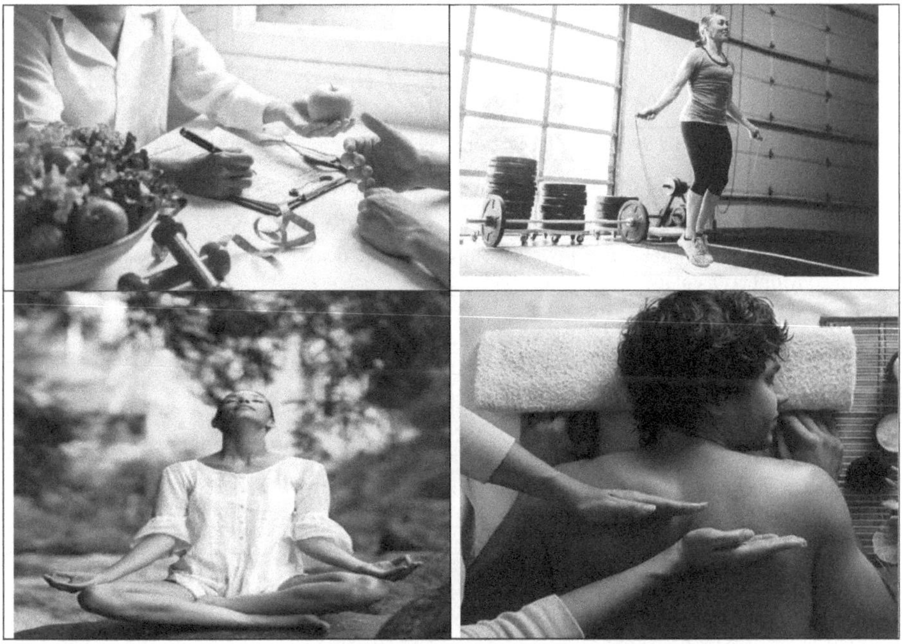

Classical Unani literature lists many potent medicines described as having:

• **Muqawwi-i-Bah** (aphrodisiac/vitalizer)
• **Muqawwi-i-Rahim** (uterine tonic)
• **Muwallid-i-Mani** (ovulation enhancer)
• **Mughalliz-i-Mani** (semen thickening agent) Common herbs/formulations include:
• **Withania somnifera, Barleria prionitis, Anogeissus latifolia, Nymphaea alba**: Used in mixtures like *Safuf Moaene Haml* or *Majun-i-Mocharas* to stimulate ovulation and uterine tone.

Usool /Principle	Purpose in Infertility
Cleanup (Tazkiyah/Imala)	Remove toxins, rebalance humors
Regimens (Tadbir)	Lifestyle/diet guidance, massage, stress control
Herbal Therapy (Dawa)	Support ovulation, uterine health, semen quality
Timing (Cycle-based)	Begin treatments around 5th day of cycle to align with ovulation window

Advise:

- **Formulations are typically timed** from day 5 of the menstrual cycle to coincide with ovulation.
- **Therapies are individualized**, depending on personal temperament (mizaj) and primary causes (e.g., anovulation, structural issues, or idiopathic infertility).
- **Approach includes multi-pronged support**—diet, detox, mental wellness, and phytopharmacology working together.

List of Unani drugs:

Withania somnifera (Asgand / Winter Cherry)

- A principal aphrodisiac and rejuvenator in Unani formulations.
- Also provides memory support (*muqawwī-e-ḥāfiẓa*), nervine strength, and anti-inflammatory effects

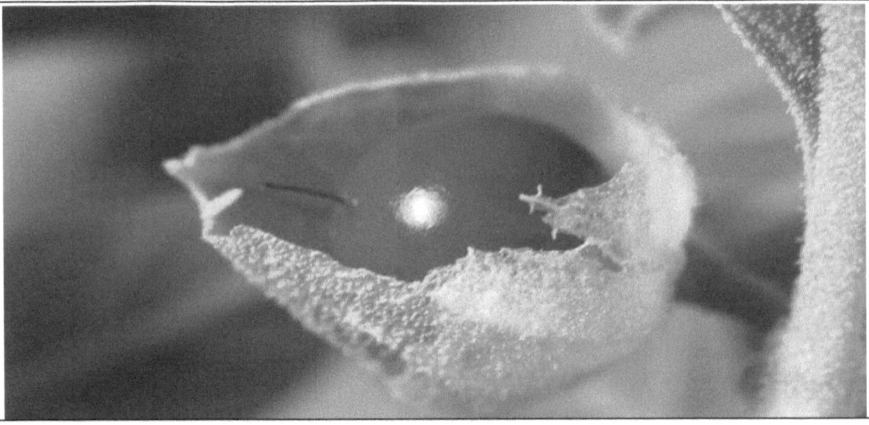

Satawar (*Asparagus racemosus*)

- Recognized for its aphrodisiac (muqawwi-e-bah), semen enhancement (*mughalliz-e-mani*), ovarian and uterine tonicity (*muqawwi-e-rahim*), and general vitality support .

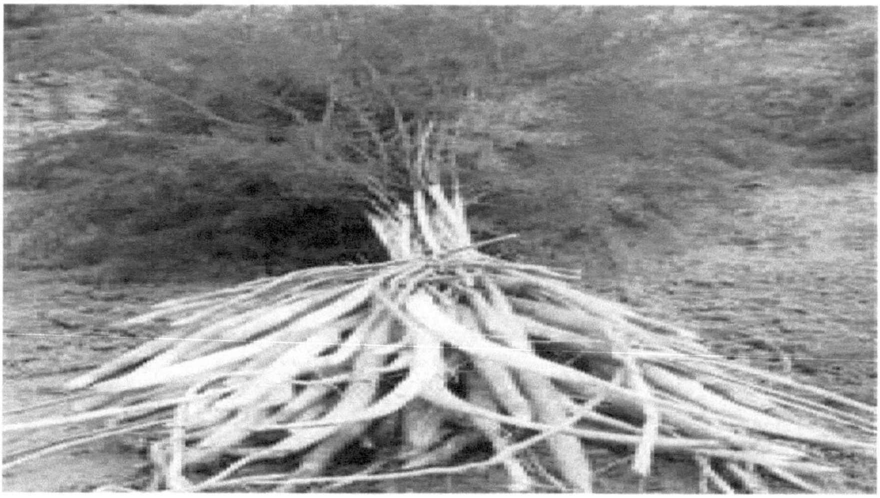

Aqarqarha (*Anacyclus pyrethrum*)

- Traditionally used to enhance libido, semen retention (*mumsik-e-mani*), general strength (*muqawwi-i-aam*), and reproductive function .

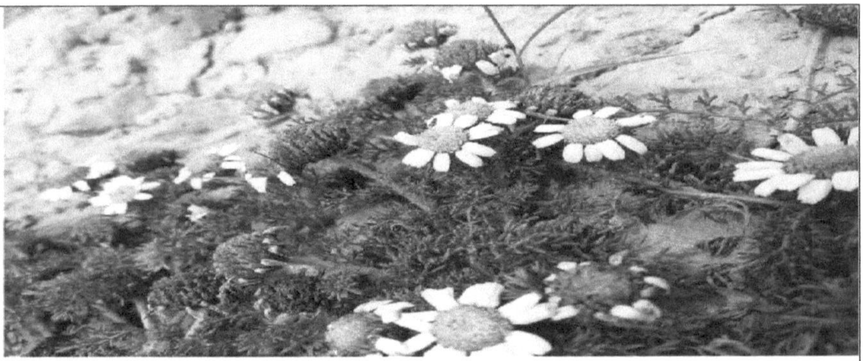

Gond keel / Khushk Gonda (Acacia resin)

•	Present in many Unani compounds like *Majūn Muqawwi Reham*.
•	Associated with uterine support and aphrodisiac properties

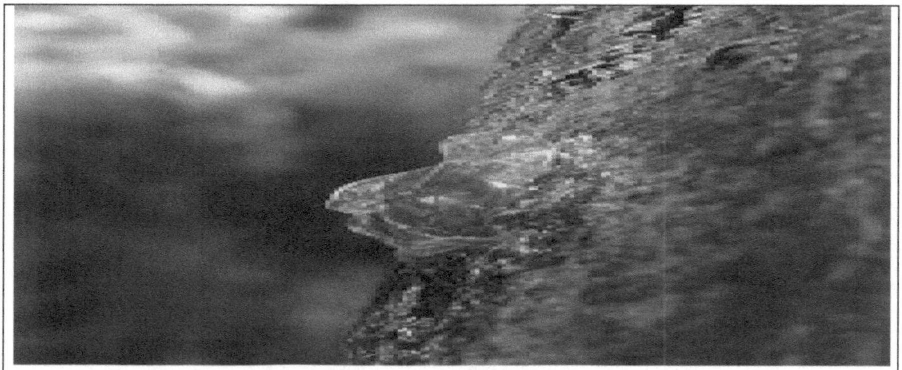

Majun Muqawwi Reham

- Formulated to tone the uterus, enhance ovulation, and support female reproductive health.
- Contains saffron, winter cherry, *satawar,* and other herbs with well-established aphrodisiac and uterine strengthening roles

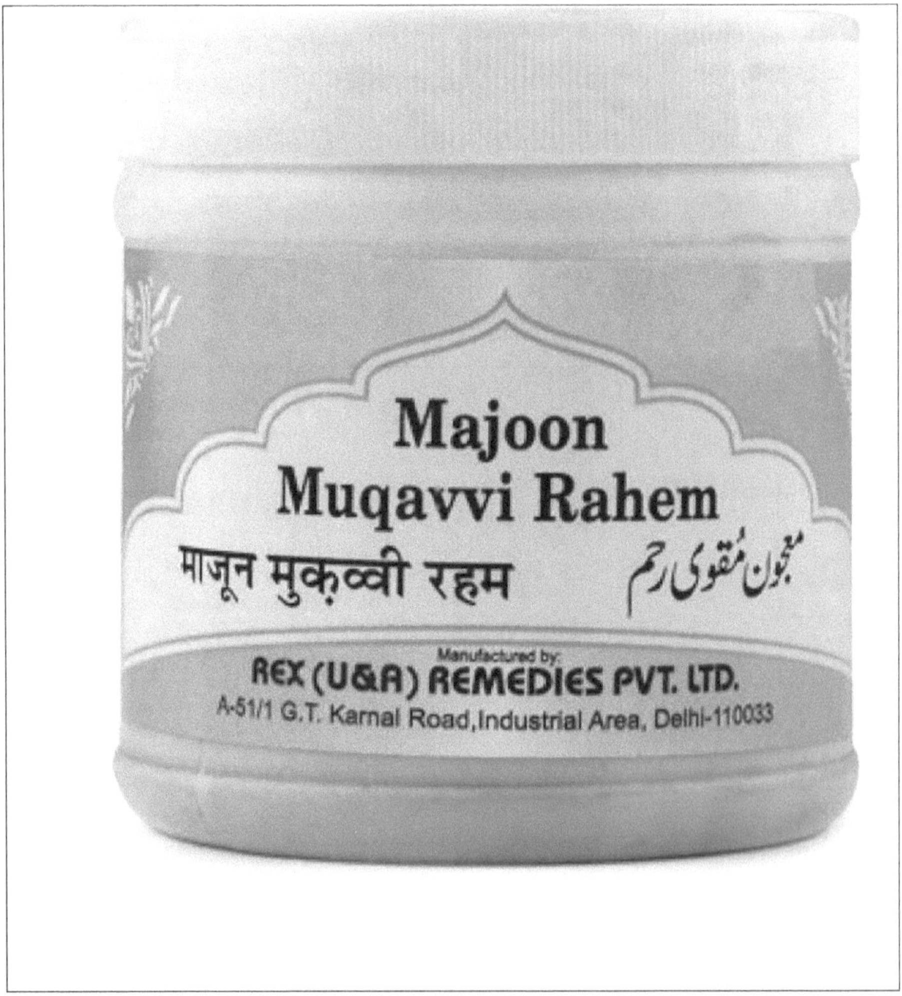

Habbe Muqawwi Khas

• Used in male reproductive weakness—supports seminal quality, libido, and nervous system vitality.
• Includes ingredients like *Asgand, saffron, Anacyclus, long pepper, pearls*, and other traditional aphrodisiacs

Drug / Formulation	Primary Muqawwi-e-Bah Use
Withania somnifera	General aphrodisiac, virility, semen quality
Asparagus racemosus	Uterine tonic, libido, semen thickener
Anacyclus pyrethrum	Male potency, semen retention, vigor
Gond keel (Acacia resin)	Potent aphrodisiac in multiple formulations
Majūn Muqawwi Reham	Female reproductive strength and fertility
Habbe Muqawwi Khas	Male sexual debility, seminal quality

Usage Considerations

• **Individualization**: Selection depends on temperament (mizāj), root cause (e.g., low semen volume, uterine weakness, libido issues), and gender.
• **Compound design**: Many classical formulations pair several of these agents to synergize aphrodisiac, uterine, and systemic tonics.
• **Professional guidance**: Accurate dosage, cycle timing, and patient temperament must be considered under supervision of a certified Unani practitioner.
• **Modern studies**: Some herbs—like *Withania somnifera, Satawar, Aqarqarha*—have shown potential in modern pharmacological research for testosterone support, anti-inflammatory action, and antioxidant benefits

Additionally, raising awareness about the impact of age on fertility can help individuals make informed decisions about family planning.

Preventions:

Maintain a Healthy Lifestyle

Balanced Diet

- Eat foods rich in antioxidants (vitamin C, E, selenium, zinc) to improve egg and sperm quality.
- Include healthy fats, whole grains, fruits, vegetables, and lean protein.
- Avoid trans fats and excessive sugar.

Maintain Healthy Weight

- **Obesity** and **underweight** conditions disrupt hormonal balance and ovulation.
- Women with PCOS and men with metabolic syndrome benefit significantly from weight management.

Regular Exercise

- Moderate physical activity improves hormonal balance, blood circulation, and stress control.
- Avoid excessive training, which can lower reproductive hormone levels.

2. Avoid Harmful Substances

No Smoking

- Smoking reduces egg and sperm quality, increases miscarriage risk, and leads to early menopause.

Limit Alcohol

- Alcohol affects ovulation in women and lowers testosterone/sperm count in men.

Avoid Recreational Drugs

- Marijuana, cocaine, and anabolic steroids can harm fertility in both genders.

3. Reduce Environmental & Occupational Hazards

Limit Exposure to:

- **Radiation & industrial chemicals** (pesticides, heavy metals like lead, solvents)
- **Heat exposure** in men (e.g., avoid hot tubs, tight underwear, prolonged laptop use on lap)
- **Endocrine disruptors** in plastics (BPA, phthalates)

4. Manage Stress & Mental Health

- Chronic stress can interfere with hormone levels and ovulation/spermatogenesis.
- Engage in yoga, meditation, mindfulness, and counseling if needed.

5. Prevent & Treat Infections

Sexually Transmitted Infections (STIs)

- STIs like **chlamydia** and **gonorrhea** can cause pelvic inflammatory disease (PID) and blocked fallopian tubes.
- **Prevention:** Use protection, get regular screenings, and treat infections early.

Reproductive Tract Infections

- Maintain genital hygiene.
- Seek prompt treatment for symptoms like discharge, pain, or abnormal bleeding.

---

6. Optimize Reproductive Health

Regular Health Checkups

- Hormonal tests, ultrasound, and semen analysis can detect early signs of infertility.
- Early detection enables prompt treatment and prevention of complications.

Track Ovulation

- For women, understanding menstrual cycles helps optimize timing of conception and detect irregularities early

7. Avoid Unnecessary Delay in Childbearing

- Fertility declines with age, especially after:
  - **35 years** in women (decline in egg quality/quantity)
  - **40+ years** in men (decline in sperm motility/DNA integrity)
- If planning to delay, consider options like **egg/sperm freezing**.

8. Avoid Unnecessary Hormonal Medications or Supplements

- Only take hormone-altering drugs or fertility supplements under medical supervision.
- Misuse can disrupt natural reproductive hormone balance.

9. Prevent Chronic Diseases or Manage Them Early

- **Diabetes, thyroid disorders, hypertension**, and autoimmune diseases can affect fertility.
- Proper control and early management reduce their impact on reproductive health.

10.In Unani Medicine: Prevention Includes

- **Maintaining balanced mizaj (temperament)**—avoid cold/dry diets and habits.
- **Use of tonics** like *Asgandh*, *Satawar*, *Qust* to strengthen reproductive organs.
- **Hijama (cupping)** and **herbal regimens** to improve blood circulation and hormonal function.
- Lifestyle modification: avoiding late-night sleep, sedentary routine, and constipation.

References:

1. Hurt, K. J., Guile, M. W., Bienstock, J. L., Fox, H. E., & Wallach, E. E. (2012). The Johns Hopkins manual of gynecology and obstetrics. Lippincott Williams & Wilkins.
2. Dc. Dutta Text book of Gynaecology.7th Ed. New Delhi: Jaypee the health sciences publishers, 2016; 17:186,188.
3. World Health organization .reproductive health indicators for global monitoring: Report of second interagency meeting, 2001.Geneva:2001.23.
4. Ibn sina .Alqanoon fil tib (Urdu translation by kantoori GH) vol VI and VIII. New Delhi:Idarekitabul shifa;2010 ;27-28,606-09.
5. Ibn-e-Hubal Baghdadi. KitabulMukhtarat fil tibb, vol I and II New Delhi : CCRUM; 2007;50-51
6. Majoosi ABA, Kamilussana (urdutransltionby Kantoorivol I and vol II,New Delhi:Idarekitabul Shifa;2010:538-540.

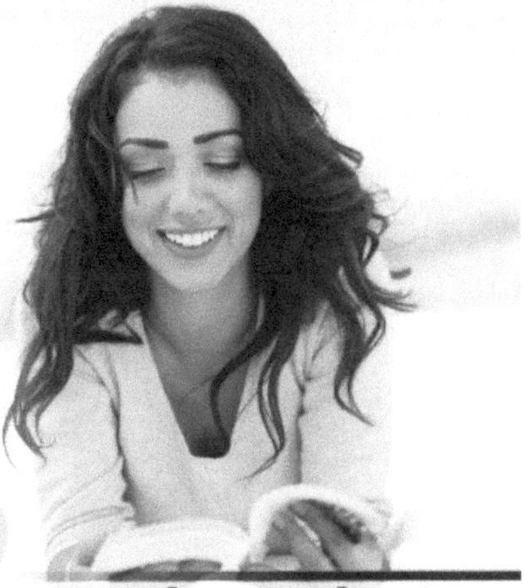

FSC
www.fsc.org
MIX
Papier | Fördert gute Waldnutzung
FSC® C083411

Kolibri 360 GmbH
Ferdinand-Jühlke-Straße 7
99095 Erfurt, Deutschland
produktsicherheit@kolibri360.de

Druck:
CPI Druckdienstleistungen GmbH
im Auftrag der
Kolibri 360 GmbH
Ferdinand-Jühlke-Str. 7
99095 Erfurt